Vegan Protein Smoothies
Superfood Vegan Smoothie Recipes for Vibrant Health, Muscle Building & Optimal Nutrition

By Karen Greenvang (aka Karen Vegan)

Copyright ©Karen Greenvang 2016

All rights reserved. No part of this publication may be reproduced, stored in a retrieval system, or transmitted, in any form or by any means, electronic, mechanical, photocopying, recording or otherwise, without the prior written permission of the author and the publishers.

The scanning, uploading, and distribution of this book via the Internet, or via any other means, without the permission of the author is illegal and punishable by law. Please purchase only authorized electronic editions, and do not participate in or encourage electronic piracy of copyrighted materials.

All information in this book has been carefully researched and checked for factual accuracy. However, the author and publishers make no warranty, expressed or implied, that the information contained herein is appropriate for every individual, situation or purpose, and assume no responsibility for errors or omission. The reader assumes the risk and full responsibility for all actions, and the author will not be held liable for any loss or damage, whether consequential, incidental, and special or otherwise, that may result from the information presented in this publication.

All cooking is an experiment in a sense, and many people come to the same or similar recipe over time. All recipes in this book have been derived from author's personal experience. Should any bear a close resemblance to those used elsewhere, that is purely coincidental.

The book is not intended to provide medical advice or to take the place of medical advice and treatment from your personal physician. Readers are advised to consult their own doctors or other qualified health professionals regarding the treatment of medical conditions. The author shall not be held liable or responsible for any misunderstanding or misuse of the information contained in this book. The information is not intended to diagnose, treat or cure any disease.

It is important to remember that the author of this book is not a doctor/ medical professional. Only opinions based upon her own personal experiences or research are cited. THE AUTHOR DOES NOT OFFER MEDICAL ADVICE or prescribe any treatments. For any health or medical issues – you should be talking to your doctor first.

Vegan Protein Smoothies

Introduction...6

Recipes...9

Peanut Butter & Banana Smoothie...9

Almond, Flaxseed & Banana Smoothie...11

Blueberry Breakfast Smoothie...13

Mango & Almond Butter Smoothie...15

Cinnamon & Apple Protein Smoothie...17

Spinach & Avocado Smoothie...19

The Green Machine Protein Smoothie...21

Pumpkin Protein Smoothie...23

The Ultimate Superfood Smoothie...24

Choc Strawberry Delight...27

Chia & Coconut Smoothie...28

Mango & Pumpkin Seed Smoothie

Protein Power Smoothie...31

Triple Chocolate Overload...32

Blueberry, Vanilla Protein Smoothie...33

Trio of Nuts Smoothie...35

Cashew & Spirulina Smoothie...37

Peach & Oats Breakfast Smoothie...39

Cashew Butter & Oatmeal Morning Glory Smoothie...41
Leafy Green Dream...43
Lime-Jalepeño Mango Protein Smoothie...44
Tropical Mint Protein Smoothie...45
Pumpkin Orange Cream Smoothie...47
Green Vegan Paleo Smoothie...49
Summer Fruits Quinoa Protein Smoothie...51
Dark Chocolate Peppermint Protein Shake...53
Carrot Cake Protein Smoothie...55
Caramel Vanilla Bean Hazelnut Milk...57
Conclusion...59

Introduction

People who adopt a vegan lifestyle are often misjudged…

Often, you'll hear critics say things like, "How can you be vegan when you can't eat anything?"

But when living a vegan lifestyle, you can still enjoy a healthy, balanced and varied diet, with the ability to enjoy many different foods, meals and beverages.

Most view the diet as being a response to animal cruelty and whilst this is a fantastic, motivating factor, another advantage of being vegan are the enormous health benefits it provides

Here are 5 benefits you'll experience from being vegan:

1. Prevention of Cardiovascular Disease

Studies have shown that adopting a vegan lifestyle can reduce the risk of type 2 diabetes and heart disease. By eliminating the unnatural dairy and meat products and eating more natural grains and nuts, people that adopt a vegan diet often experience increases in their cardiovascular health.

2. Weight Loss & Increased Energy

Natural weight loss is often a by-product of living a vegan lifestyle. A vegan diet eliminates most of the unhealthy, processed foods that contribute to weight gain and obesity. By avoiding foods high in saturated fat and sugar, whilst consuming healthier, natural foods like nuts, fruits & vegetables, vegans not only lose fat, but also experience an increase in energy. The avoidance is processed sugar is a big factor in a person's energy levels.

3. Avoiding Cow's Milk

Did you know that humans are the only species that continues to drink milk after childhood? Milk is not designed to be consumed into adult life and most adults are lactose intolerant or have milk allergies and don't know it. Vegan's drink healthier alternatives, such as almond milk or rice milk, which have added health benefits.

4. Eliminating the Risk of Salmonella & Mad Cow Disease

The deadly infection Salmonella, as well as Mad Cow Disease, are both illnesses brought on by eating animal products. The virus is usually contracted when a person comes into contact with raw eggs or raw chicken. Eliminating these foods from your diet means there is no risk of contracting the illnesses.

5. Healthy Skin & a Longer Life

The vitamins found in nuts and vegetables contribute to healthy and glowing skin. So, those who eat a vegan diet will experience an improvement in this area. Studies have also shown that vegans & vegetarians often live longer than those who are not. These benefits to health contribute to vegans having more energy, healthier skin, nails and hair and living longer by preventing major diseases.

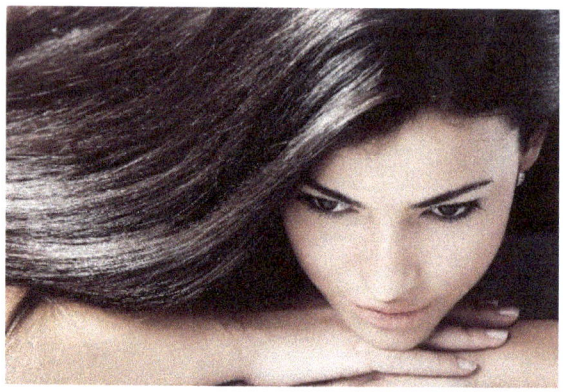

Amazing Vegan Smoothie Recipes That Are Naturally Rich in Protein

Peanut Butter & Banana Smoothie

This recipe contains two of the healthiest and tastiest ingredients you can use in a vegan Smoothie – peanut butter and bananas! The bananas are high in potassium, vitamin B6 and Vitamin C, while the peanut butter is an excellent source of protein. Infact, peanut butter is one of the best vegan sources of protein and should be featured in many of your vegan smoothies.

The bananas are best used frozen and I find the best way to freeze them for easy use is to cut them up into small slices, then spread them out on an oven tray with a sheet of baking paper on top. This way they will be easy to grab from the freezer and throw in the blender when you're ready to go! This smoothie tastes amazing and is packed with protein to give you an energy boost.

Serves: 1-2

Ingredients:

- 2 bananas, sliced
- 3 small pitted dates
- 1 heaped tbsp. of peanut butter
- ¾ cup of almond milk

Directions:

1. Place all ingredients in a high-power blender.
2. Blend until smooth and combined (if the mixture is too thick, you can add a small amount of water to thin out the mixture).
3. Serve into a chilled glass.

Almond, Flaxseed & Banana Smoothie

The banana makes yet another appearance, as it is a great fruit with amazing health benefits and great qualities for making a tasty, thick smoothie. Almonds are another great source of protein and are also low in saturated fats. Using almonds in this recipe as well as almond milk provides a healthy and high-protein shake.

The flaxseed meal is an excellent source of Omega-3 fatty acids, aka 'good fats'. Good fats are also found in almonds, so this smoothie is packed full of both healthy fats and protein. After having this smoothie, not only will you feel full and satisfied but you will also get an energy boost from the banana's and natural source of protein. Peach makes it taste great!

Serves: 1-2

Ingredients:

- 2 bananas, sliced
- 15-20 almonds
- 1 big peach
- ¾ cup of almond milk,
- 2 tsp. of flaxseed meal

Directions:

1. Place all ingredients in a high-power blender.

2. Blend until combined and almonds are blitzed.
3. Serve into a chilled glass.

Tip: Add a small amount of water or coconut water (fantastic after workouts) if you want a thinner smoothie.

Blueberry Breakfast Smoothie

This blueberry breakfast smoothie is the perfect way to start your morning. It can be used as a meal replacement for your normal breakfast, as the ingredients used will provide you with enough nutrients and energy to keep you active and alert all day. If you're in a rush, sleep in or aren't usually a breakfast eater – then this smoothie will change your life! It's easy to prepare and will keep you going all day.

It provides a great slow release of energy from the oats, antioxidants and essential nutrients from the blueberries. It's thick, delicious and will make you feel full until your next meal.

Ingredients:

- 1 cup of almond milk
- ½ cup of fresh blueberries
- 2 tbsp. of gluten-free oats
- 1 tsp. of vanilla extract
- 1 tbsp. of hemp seeds
- 1 tbsp. chia seeds

Directions:

1. Add almond milk, oats, vanilla, hemp seeds and chia seeds to a high-powered blender.
2. Then, add the blueberries and blitz until well combined.
3. Pour into a chilled glass and serve. You can also use it to make a smoothie bowl- I love it before my workouts. Top it up with more nuts and seeds to create an amazing vegan energy breakfast!

Mango & Almond Butter Smoothie

It's no secret by now that nut butters are an excellent source of protein. Almond butter is high in protein, low in saturated fat and has a great taste. The almond butter gives this smoothie a thick, creamy texture making it taste amazing and is very filling. Mangoes are also a fantastic source of important vitamins that will help you stay energized and alert.

Try to avoid the bigger brands that are found in the spreads aisle and instead buy from an organic source in the health foods section. They cost a bit extra but it is definitely worth it.

This recipe also includes rice malt syrup, which is an alternative to maple syrup that is sourced from brown rice. It is a healthier option, as maple syrup often contains processed sugars, the rice malt syrup provides the same consistency and a similar flavour whilst also providing the health benefits of a complex carbohydrate.

Serves: 1-2

Ingredients:

- 2 cups of mango, cut into chunks
- ¼ cup of almond butter
- ½ cup of almond milk
- 1/3 cup of rice malt syrup
- A dash of water
- Mint leaves (optional)

Directions:

1. Add mango, almond butter, almond milk and rice malt syrup to a high-powered blender.
2. Blend together until well combined.
3. If needed, add a dash of water to thin the mixture.
4. Pour into a chilled glass, garnish with some mint leaves and serve.

Cinnamon & Apple Protein Smoothie

This is an incredibly delicious smoothie that can be used as a breakfast replacement if you are on the go. Cinnamon & apple is a classic flavour combination and when combined in this smoothie provides a great source of protein and vitamins. The main source of protein from this smoothie is from the oats and the almond butter. The apple provides a great hit of energy and the oats will provide enough protein and fibre to keep you full & satisfied as well as energies for the rest of the morning or afternoon.

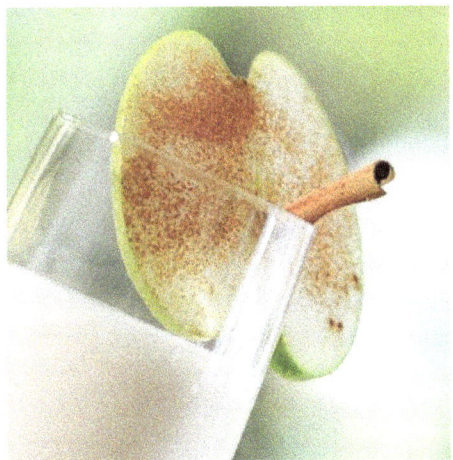

You can also use the apple peel in this recipe. The peel holds the greatest concentration of vitamins so it is a great benefit if you include it.

Serves: 1-2

Ingredients:

- 1 apple, sliced
- ½ cup of gluten-free oats
- ½ tsp. of cinnamon
- 1 tbsp. of almond butter
- ½ cup of almond milk
- A dash of water

Directions:

1. Add the almond milk and oats to a high-powered blender.
2. Pulse until well combined. Allow to rest for 2-3 minutes.
3. Add the rest of the ingredients to the blender and blitz until well combined.
4. Pour into a chilled glass and serve.

Spinach & Avocado Smoothie

This savoury smoothie recipe packs its secret punch of protein from hulled hemp seeds. Hulled hemp seeds can be purchased in the healthy foods section of your local super market and are an incredible natural source of protein. Spinach is also a great all-rounder in smoothie recipes, blends easy, proteins an extra bit of protein and doesn't affect the flavour of the beverage at all.

Avocado is also a great ingredient to use in smoothies and other vegan recipes. It is super high in healthy fats and can be used as a spread, in smoothies or in a salad. This is a great green smoothie recipe that can be drunk at any time of the day. It provides a boost of energy to help get you through the rest of the day.

Serves: 2

Ingredients:

- 1 cup almond milk
- 1 cup spinach leaves
- ½ cucumber, chopped
- 1 tbsp. of avocado
- 2 large pitted dates

Directions:

1. Add all ingredients to a high-powered blender.
2. Blitz until well combined.
3. Pour into a chilled glass and serve.

The Green Machine Protein Smoothie

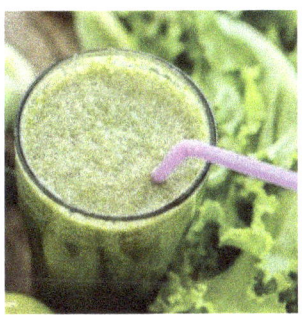

Here is an overview of all the greens you'll find in this vegan smoothie, along with the health benefits you'll gain from including them in your diet. The king of the greens found in this smoothie recipe is spinach. The hipsters of today are obsessed with Kale (don't get me wrong- I like kale as well) but spinach certainly rivals it and may even surpass it in terms of health benefits.

Spinach in packed full of iron (more than you will find in a T-bone steak) and has also been found to work as an appetite suppressant. If you drink this smoothie first thing in the morning, chances are you'll feel full for longer and it will help you lose weight!

Chard is packed full of anti-inflammatory antioxidants and studies have shown that it can help to prevent type 2 diabetes. This little known leafy green doesn't have the mainstream fame of kale or spinach, but including this vegetable in your diet will be a huge benefit to your health.

Water retention is a condition where the body holds more water than it should. The tissues absorb extra water and this can lead to complications and possible kidney disease, heart failure, lung disease and arthritis. The next two greens that are found in this recipe both help to prevent water retention, making them important players in this green machine smoothie!

Firstly, celery is a great source of fibre and B vitamins and will also contribute to the prevention of water retention. Cucumber is also packed full of fibre and B vitamins and will also join the fight against water retention. Cucumber is also a great source of electrolytes to give you a welcome energy boost.

Dubbed 'the beauty food', Watercress is the secret weapon in this green machine, protein-packed smoothie. Watercress is the leader of anti-aging vegetables, with enormous amounts of vitamin K and other healthy nutrients that contribute to healthy skin, hair and nails. If you want to look and feel younger, you need to start adding watercress to your diet and of course to your smoothies! Studies have also shown that watercress can help prevent cancer. Just another reason to add it to your smoothie every day!

Serves: 2

Ingredients:

- 1 cup spinach
- 1 cup cucumber, chopped
- ½ cup of celery, chopped
- ½ cup of fresh watercress
- 1 chard leaf
- ½ cup of almond milk

Directions:

1. Add all Ingredients to a high-powered blender and blitz until well combined.

Pumpkin Protein Smoothie

If you are looking from a break from the regular green vegan smoothies, this pumpkin smoothie is a great alternative. The pumpkin adds a filling flavour as well as a huge dose of vitamin A, which has a range of health benefits including healthier teeth, bones and blood cells.

The pumpkin protein smoothie is super easy to make and is a great option at any time of the day. Make sure you use an organic pumpkin puree to ensure it's the best quality and is vegan-friendly.

Serves: 1-2

Ingredients:

- 1 cup of almond milk
- ½ cup of organic pumpkin puree
- 1 tbsp. of organic almond butter
- ½ tsp. of cinnamon powder
- Small handful of hemp seeds, optional

Directions:

1. Add all ingredients to a high-powered blender.
2. Blitz until well combined.
3. Pour into a chilled glass and serve.

The Ultimate Superfood Smoothie

This superfood smoothie packs a protein punch as well as providing an array of benefits from the different superfoods used in the recipe. It will keep you energized for the most of the day and will help fight off those mid-morning cravings. Here is a list of the superfoods in this recipe, as well as the health benefits they provide:

Cacao Nibs – they are high in fibre, magnesium and iron. Magnesium is responsible for muscle and nerve function and help keeps hearth rhythm steady. Iron is necessary for red blood cell production and fibre is essential for healthy digestion. Cacao nibs are also a much healthier alternative to dark chocolate!

Maca Powder – is a root that belongs to the Radish family, and should be a popular superfood powder in every vegan's pantry. Maca powder is rich in vitamins B, C & E, as well as zinc, iron and magnesium. The antioxidants found in maca powder have also been shown to boost your mood, provide more energy and give you healthier skin.

Flaxseed Meal – This ingredient has featured in a previous recipe, and is very high in healthy omega-3 fatty acids. These good fats have been shown to have a positive impact on heart health and can help to prevent heart disease and cardiovascular disease. Packed full of antioxidants and fibre, some recent studies have shown the Flaxseed may help lower the risk of breast cancer, prostate cancer and colon cancer.

Chia Seeds – Chia seeds are another excellent source of healthy omega-3 fats. Another benefit of these healthy fats is that they raise HDL cholesterol levels, which is the good cholesterol that helps fight against heart and lung disease. They are also high in fibre, magnesium, vitamin B3, calcium, zinc and many other important nutrients.

Hemp Seeds – Hemp seeds are yet another excellent vegan source of healthy omega-3 fatty acids. What makes hemp seeds stand out from the others though, is the fact that it also boasts a good amount of protein. Adding hemp seeds to any smoothie is a great way to add an extra hit of protein to your drink.

Goji Berries – Goji berries contain a great amount of antioxidants that help to give you healthy skin and protect the eyes. They also help to boost your immune system. They also provide a source of complex carbohydrates which will ensure you have a sustained release of energy, helping you to keep active throughout the entire day.

Serves: 1-2

Ingredients:

- 1 ½ cups of rice milk
- 1 banana
- 2 tbsp. of cacao nibs
- 1 tbsp. of maca powder
- 2 tsp. of flaxseed meal
- 1 tbsp. of chia seeds
- 1 tsp. of hemp seeds
- 1 tsp. of vanilla extract
- A small handful of goji berries, to garnish

Directions:

1. Add rice milk, banana, cacao nibs, maca powder, flaxseed meal, chia seeds, and hemp seeds into a high-powered blender.
2. Blitz until well combined.
3. Pour into a chilled glass.
4. Sprinkle Goji Berries or other fruits on top and serve.

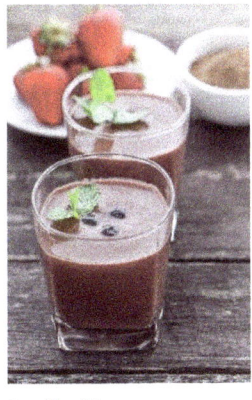
Choc Strawberry Delight

This chocolate and strawberry flavoured smoothie not only tastes amazing, but it provides a huge range of health benefits thanks to the superfoods that are included in the recipe. Strawberries have a huge range of healthy nutrients and vitamins including magnesium, phosphorus, potassium, iodine, folate, dietary fibre, vitamin B6, biotin and omega-3 fatty acids.

They are an excellent option for your smoothie and your vegan diet in general, as the health benefits they provide are incredible.

Serves: 2

Ingredients:

- 1 cup of coconut milk
- 1 cup of organic strawberries
- 1 tbsp. of cacao nibs
- 1 tbsp. of hemp seeds
- 1 tbsp. of chia seeds
- A small handful of raw almonds

Directions:

1. Add all ingredients into a high-powered blender.
2. Blitz until well combined and Ice Cubes are dissolved.
3. Pour into a chilled glass and serve.

Chia & Coconut Smoothie

If you aren't a fan of almond milk or you just want to mix things up, then coconut milk is another great option for a dairy free, vegan-friendly milk source. Coconuts are an excellent source of B vitamins, as well as A & E, iron, magnesium, calcium and sodium.

Chia seeds will give you a boost of energy and provide you with essential omega-3 fatty acids, while the protein source will be provided by the tofu.

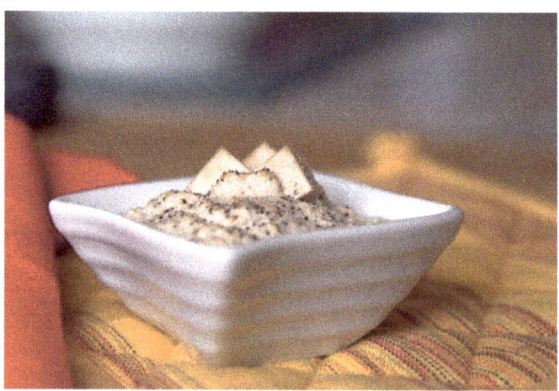

Tofu is one of the best sources you can find for protein that is vegan-friendly and this smoothie is a fantastic, tasty and super easy recipe for when you want a quick energy hit.

Serves: 1-2

Ingredients:

- 1 cup of coconut milk
- 4 tbsp. desiccated coconut
- ½ cup of water
- ½ of a banana, sliced
- 1 tbsp. chia seeds

- ¼ cup tofu
- Some fruits (for example strawberries to garnish)

Directions:

1. Add all ingredients into a high-powered blender.
2. Blitz until well combined.
3. Pour into a chilled glass, garnish with fruits of your choice and serve.

Tip: If the smoothie is too thick, add a small amount of water to the mixture and blend until it has reached your desired consistency.

Mango & Pumpkin Seed Smoothie

Perfect for a hot summer's day. The mango is one of those fruits that instantly makes you think of summer. When summer rolls around and mangoes are in season, there's nothing better than enjoying one in the sun and coupled with pumpkin seeds, this smoothie will not only quench your thirst and cool you down, but it will give you a mood and energy boost and have you energized and excited for the rest of the sunny day! But if it is a hot day and you are looking for a delicious smoothie that isn't too filling but will cool you down, then pumpkin seeds are a great source of natural high protein.

Serves: 1-2

Ingredients:

- 1 cup of coconut milk
- 1 cup of mango, cut into chunks
- 2 tbsp. of pumpkin seeds
- 1 tbsp. of coconut oil

Directions:

1. Add all ingredients to a high-powered blender.
2. Blitz until well combined.
3. Pour into a chilled glass and serve.

Protein Power Smoothie

We recommend using 2 tablespoons of sunflower seeds, but feel free to add an extra one if you really want a serious protein hit. This smoothie is great after a session at the gym, as it's a great way to help your muscles recovery quicker. The raw almonds are a great source of omega-3 fatty acids, and along with the banana, will help to replace some of that energy burnt off in the gym.

Ingredients:

- 1 cup of coconut milk
- 2 tbsp. of sunflower seeds
- 1 banana, sliced
- A small handful of raw almonds

Directions:
1. Add all ingredients to a high-powered blender.
2. Blitz until well combined.
3. Pour into a chilled glass and serve.

Triple Chocolate Overload

Chocolate lovers this is for you! And let's face it, who doesn't love indulging in chocolate? This recipe is appropriately named the 'Triple Chocolate Overload' as it gets its chocolate flavour from two different sources – Cacao nibs and cacao powder. The Banana and Almond Milk and there to provide a great consistency and a hit of energy, but let's not worry about that, because this one is all about the Chocolate!

Serves: 1-2

Ingredients:

- 1 cup of almond milk
- 1 banana, frozen and sliced
- 1 tbsp. of cacao nibs, or similar (for example raw, dark chocolate)
- 2 tsp. of cacao powder

Directions:

1. Add all ingredients into a high-powered blender.
2. Blend until well combined.
3. Pour into a chilled glass and serve.

Tip: If the smoothie is too thick, add a small amount of water to the mixture and blend until it has reached your desired consistency.

Blueberry, Vanilla Protein Smoothie

Blueberries are an excellent source of antioxidants, and are a great option for vegan friendly smoothies. They also pair excellently with coconut milk and almond butter, making this smoothie a healthy, flavoursome option for your repertoire. This is an excellent smoothie to have first thing in the morning, as the blueberries and almond Butter will give you a much needed energy boost to help you kick start your day.

If you are feeling adventurous, you can also add spinach or even oats to this recipe to make it even more flavoursome and healthier. The spinach doesn't affect the flavour at all and the oats will provide a source of complex carbohydrate for a sustained, long lasting energy release throughout the day. This smoothie is an excellent choice if you want to skip breakfast but still feel energized and full when you walk out the door ready to start your day!

Serves: 1-2

Ingredients:

- 1 cup of coconut milk
- ½ cup of blueberries
- 1 tbsp. of almond butter
- 1 tbsp. vanilla powder
- 5 tbsp. organic oats, soaked in water

Directions:

1. Add all ingredients into a high-powered blender.
2. Blend until well combined.
3. Pour into a chilled glass and serve.

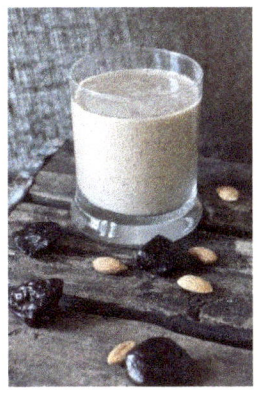
Trio of Nuts Smoothie

If you love nuts, then you'll go nuts for this smoothie. Nuts are nut butters are probably one of my favourite foods. They taste great, and the health benefits are almost endless. They provide a great source of healthy fats as well as being one of the best natural vegan sources of protein. They each have unique, delicious flavours, and when combined in the following recipe they taste amazing.

This smoothie is all about the nut. It uses three different types of nuts (almonds, walnuts and peanuts), and from three different sources (milk, butter and raw). It is an excellent treat to have post-dinner or just after lunch. If you want to change the consistency of the smoothie, try adding some extra water to make it thinner, or if you'd prefer a thicker smoothie, try adding an extra scoop of either nut Butter.

Serves: 2

Ingredients:

- 1 cup of almond milk
- ½ cup of water
- ½ cup of almond butter
- ½ cup of peanut butter
- A small handful of raw almonds
- A small handful of raw walnuts
- 1 banana, sliced and frozen

Directions:

1. Add all ingredients to a high-powered blender.
2. Blitz until well combined
3. Pour into a chilled glass and serve.

Tip: If the smoothie is too thick, add a small amount of water to the mixture and blend until it has reached your desired consistency.

Cashew & Spirulina Smoothie

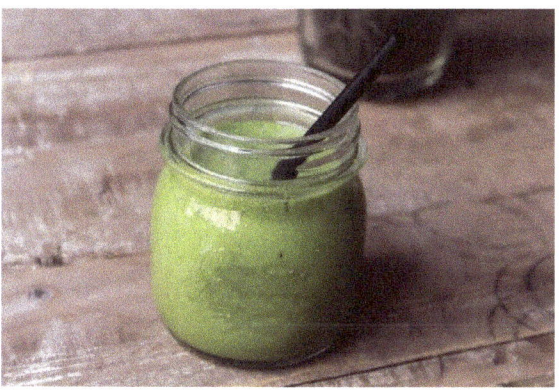

Another member of the nut family that is one of the best sources of protein is the cashew. Cashews are very rich and textured. They are delicious and I often find myself and handful after handful of cashews in between meals. They also work great in smoothies, cashew and cinnamon works great together.

Spirulina powder is another impressively beneficial member of the superfood family. It also boasts incredible health benefits such as vitamins B, C, D, E, A, potassium, copper, iron and calcium. I know a lot of people who absolutely love spirulina and swear by it, but I find that it can be a little bitter if you use too much. Therefore, I try to use it sparingly (as shown is this recipe), so that it doesn't over power the rest of the ingredients.

If you're not a big fan of spirulina, you can try replacing it with maca powder or hemp seeds. Using hemp seeds will give you an extra dose of protein for those post-work out smoothies.

Serves: 1-2

Ingredients:

- Handful of blueberries
- 1 cup of coconut milk
- ½ cup of raw cashews
- 1 tbsp. of spirulina powder
- 1 tsp. of cinnamon powder

Directions:

1. Add all ingredients to a high-powered blender.
2. Blitz until well combined.
3. Pour into a chilled glass and serve.

Peach & Oats Breakfast Smoothie

Who doesn't love the combination of peaches and oats in their morning breakfast? The peach is one of my all-time favourite fruits, it's absolutely delicious and goes tremendously well with oats in the morning. I would religiously eat peach & cooked oats for breakfast every morning, until I discovered this recipe. It uses the same ingredients (plus a few extras for added benefit) and gives you a big boost of energy in the morning. Not only that but it tastes even better than the morning oats I always use to have!

The fact that you can blend these amazing, healthy ingredients together and enjoy a delicious smoothie packed full of nutrients every morning is convenient and delightful. You'll also get yourself a great hit of protein thanks to the hemp seeds and rolled oats. If organic peaches are in season at your local super market, make the most of it and try out this fantastic morning recipe!

Serves: 1-2

Ingredients:

- 1-2 peaches, quartered with pits removed
- ¾ cup of almond milk
- ½ cup of rolled oats
- ½ cup of hemp seeds
- A dash of water, optional

Directions:

1. Add all ingredients to a high-powered blender.
2. Blitz until well combined.
3. Pour into a chilled glass and serve.

Cashew Butter & Oatmeal Morning Glory Smoothie

The title for this smoothie says it all. Once you've tried this recipe you'll literally bounce out of bed in anticipation ready to drink this incredibly delicious smoothie. Not only does it taste heavenly, but it is super packed with protein from the peanut butter and oatmeal. I've given it the name the 'morning glory smoothie' because I've found it to be such an effective mood booster, possibly due to the fact that peanut butter is one of my all-time favourites.

The hemp seeds are optional, I usually don't add hemp seeds, but if you're looking to get more protein into your diet then the watermelon seeds are a great way to do this. The morning glory smoothie will also provide complex carbohydrates from the oats, so you will get a sustained, slow release of energy throughout the morning. I'm often full of energy right through until lunch time when I drink this smoothie, with no cravings for snacks in between.

Serves: 1-2

Ingredients:

- 1 cup of rice milk
- ½ cup of cashew butter
- ½ cup of rolled oats (soak in rice milk overnight for a better result)
- 1 tbsp. of watermelon seeds, optional (for an extra protein hit)
- A dash of water, optional

Directions:

1. Add all ingredients to a high-powered blender.
2. Blitz until well combined.
3. Pour into a chilled glass and serve.

Leafy Green Dream

Those of you who can't get enough of your healthy leafy greens, this recipe is for you! Leafy greens are extremely healthy sources of beneficial nutrients and antioxidants. Including leafy greens in your diet helps to aid digestion and can help with energy levels by eradicating fatigue. If you are looking to add protein to your diet, leafy greens also play an important role as they help to metabolize protein in the body. Making the most of all the best leafy green sources, the leafy green dream smoothie will have you energized and fighting fit!

Serves: 1-2

Ingredients:

- 1 cup of almond milk
- ½ cucumber, chopped
- ½ cup of spinach leaves
- ½ cup of kale
- 2-3 leafs of chard
- 2-3 leafs of romaine lettuce

Directions:

1. Add all ingredients into a high-powered blender.
2. Blitz until well combined.
3. Pour into a chilled glass and serve.

Lime-Jalepeño Mango Protein Smoothie

Counting up the protein you get from the fruits as well as the hefty dose from the seeds, this smoothie packs a total of 14.5 grams of protein in this refreshing, sweet smoothie recipe with a spicy bite. If you're looking for a creamier texture and an addition of healthy fats, you can add half an avocado. That will add about 2 more grams of protein along with about 5 grams of fibre and a bucket load of potassium, as well as other nutrients, plus a smooth, mild flavour. You just can't go wrong by adding avocado to a smoothie! You can also serve it as a raw soup- season it with Himalaya salt and you're good to go!

Serves: 1-2

Ingredients:

- 1 cup of coconut milk
- 1/2 lime, freshly squeezed
- 1 heaped tbsp. chopped jalepeño
- 1 tbsp. flaxseed, ground
- 2 tbsp. hemp seed, ground
- 1 tbsp. chia seeds, ground
- 1/2 avocado

Directions:

1. Add all ingredients into a high-powered blender.
2. Blitz until well combined.
3. Pour into a chilled glass and serve.

Tropical Mint Protein Smoothie

This is your all-day smoothie. If you have this filling meal for breakfast, you'll have energy the entire morning thanks to the fruit, and you won't want or need another meal until well into the afternoon thanks to the protein boost from the seeds. You'll get the nutrients but allow the wonderful fruit and mint flavours to help you feel refreshed all day. Acai berry puree packets are a great addition to keep handy and add to smoothies like these, but if you prefer just a simple mango, then that works great too.

Serves: 1-2

Ingredients:

- 1 large fresh orange
- ½ cup coconut milk
- 1/2 cups frozen mango
- 1 tbsp. ground flaxseeds
- 2 tbsp. ground hemp seeds
- 1 tbsp. ground chia seeds
- 4-5 fresh mint leaves
- 1 packet frozen Acai puree (optional)

Directions:

1. Add all ingredients into a high-powered blender.
2. Blitz until well combined.
3. Pour into a chilled glass and serve.

Pumpkin Orange Cream Smoothie

Do you find yourself drudging through your work day? Maybe the 2pm energy crash is a bit too familiar? The orange juice will help to revitalize with its vitamin C content, the ginger will relieve any inflammation in the body and will act as an energizer...

My favourite way to boost my spirits on a cold winter afternoon and sip on a healthy, refreshing drink.

Serves: 1-2

Ingredients:

- 1 medium orange, peeled and sliced
- 1/2 cup unsweetened orange juice
- A splash of vanilla extract
- 1/2 cup canned pumpkin puree
- 1/2 cup vanilla non-dairy yogurt
- 1 tbsp. maple syrup or stevia- optional
- 1 tbsp. grated ginger
- 1 tbsp. freshly ground flax seed

- 1/4 tsp. ground cinnamon

Directions:

1. Add all ingredients into a high-powered blender.
2. Blitz until well combined.
3. Pour into a chilled glass and serve.

Green Vegan Paleo Smoothie

This is a citrus and creamy wake me up smoothie, guaranteed to get you up and ready to go within seconds of drinking it. You'll get your daily boost of protein from the coconut cream and milk. Not to mention the sweetness from the mango and lime to give you that extra zing. The kiwi has an extremely high vitamin C content which will help fight any infections in the body and not to mention, spinach; a powerful superfood that will keep you young and glowing.

Serves: 1-2

Ingredients:

- 1 mango (diced)
- 2 cups kale (stems removed)
- 1 lime (juiced)
- 1 kiwi (diced)
- Handful of spinach
- 1 cup of coconut milk

- A dash of coconut cream (for extra thickness)
- Water

Directions:

1. Add all ingredients into a high-powered blender.
2. Blitz until well combined.
3. Pour into a chilled glass and serve.

Summer Fruits Quinoa Protein Smoothie

Did you know chia seeds contain some of the best Omega-3's found in plant form? In fact, chia seeds have more Omega-3 content than salmon, which is a true superfood.

Quinoa, another great source, is a complete protein, but it is also a prime source of magnesium, fibre and iron too. The ingredients go so well together with the mixed berries and thick coconut cream.

Serves: 1-2

Ingredients:

- 1-1/2 cups vanilla almond milk
- ¼ cup coconut cream
- 1/2 cup cooked quinoa, cooled
- 1 tbsp. chia seeds
- 1 tbsp. wheat germ

- 2 tbsp. maple syrup, stevia or other vegan sweetener- optional
- 2 cups frozen mixed berries

Directions:

1. Add all ingredients into a high-powered blender.
2. Blitz until well combined.
3. Pour into a chilled glass and serve.

Dark Chocolate Peppermint Protein Shake

Between the cocoa powder and the dark chocolate protein powder, chocolate lovers are going to want to drink this morning, noon and night. Which is absolutely fine, as dark chocolate contains a high amount of antioxidants and can help with stress regulation.

Soy sprouts powder is derived from natural plant sources and is very nutritious. This protein powder is very easily accessible and can be found in health food stores or online.

Serves: 1-2

Ingredients:

- 1 cup non-dairy milk of choice (I recommend chia seed milk for this one)
- 1 large banana, frozen
- 2 tbsp. dark cocoa powder
- 1 scoop soy sprouts powder
- 1/4 tsp. pure peppermint extract

- Pinch Himalayan sea salt

Directions:

1. Add all ingredients into a high-powered blender.
2. Blitz until well combined.
3. Pour into a chilled glass and serve.

Carrot Cake Protein Smoothie

For a dessert that won't undo a workout, blend almond milk, carrot juice, a banana, and sugar's healthy swap, cinnamon with a handful of cashews for a protein and vitamin E boost. Then sip. Aaaahh. And although it has the carrot cake flavour, it's much healthier than cake.

The cumin and cinnamon will give it that cakey taste, as well as providing you with the same benefits the Indians have been enjoying for centuries.

Serves: 1-2

Ingredients:

- ¾ cup vanilla almond milk
- ½ cup carrot juice
- 1 frozen banana
- Handful cashew nuts
- ⅛ tsp. cinnamon
- ⅛ tsp. cumin

Directions:

1. Add all ingredients into a high-powered blender.
2. Blitz until well combined.
3. Pour into a chilled glass and serve.

Caramel Vanilla Bean Hazelnut Milk

Luxurious, rich and absolutely splurge-worthy, this is a homemade hazelnut milk that is fit for a coffee shop and can be a great addition to your cappuccinos or black teas. This recipe uses a mix of soaked almonds and hazelnuts, but you can use just hazelnuts if you prefer. The flavour is caramelized with the addition of the Medjool dates, whole vanilla bean and cinnamon and you can turn it into a chocolate hazelnut milk quite easily by adding some organic dark cocoa powder. The possibilities are endless...

Serves: 1-2

Ingredients:

- 1 vanilla bean, roughly chopped
- 1/4 cup raw almonds
- 3/4 cup raw hazelnuts
- Halved 3 pitted Medjool dates, to taste

- 3 1/2 cups water
- 1/2 teaspoon cinnamon
- Pinch Himalayan salt

Directions:
1. Place hazelnuts and almonds in a bowl and cover with water. It's better to soak them overnight but you can get away with 1-2 hours.

2. Rinse and drain the soaked almonds and hazelnuts. Place nuts into a blender along with vanilla bean, pitted dates, water, cinnamon and salt.

3. Cover and blend for about a minute or until smooth

4. Place a nut milk bag (or a water separator bag) over a large bowl and slowly pour the blended mixture into the bag and gently squeeze the bottom to release the milk. Patience is key here. In the end you should be left with about 1 cup of pulp in the bag.

5. Rinse out blender and pour the milk back in. Now, pour it easily into a Mason jar and secure with lid. Chill in the fridge. Give the jar a good shake before drinking.

6. There are many ways you can use this smoothie, you can either drink it on its own, use it in cereals or add it to your oatmeal breakfast and as a creamer for your teas or coffees.

Conclusion

Thank you for reading!

I hope that with so many vegan-friendly recipes you will be motivated and inspired to start your journey towards meaningful veganism, vibrant health and total wellbeing.

Remember, the beauty of incorporating nutritious vegan foods into your daily diet is that you are making simple, yet sustainable changes that will work for your wellness long-term. Not to mention your spiritual wellness and taking care of the environment.

If you enjoyed my book, it would be greatly appreciated if you left a review so others can receive the same benefits you have. Your review can help other people take this important step to take care of their health and inspire them to start a new chapter in their lives.

At the same time, <u>you can help me serve you and all my other readers</u> even more through my next vegan-friendly recipe books that I am committed to publishing on a regular basis.

I'd be thrilled to hear from you. I would love to know your favorite recipe(s).

Don't be shy, post a comment on Amazon!

Thank You for your time,

Love & Light,

Until next time-

Karen Vegan Greenvang

Join Karen's Vegan Email Newsletter:

www.YourWellnessBooks.com/karen

It's free and every week you will be getting new awesome tips and recipes to help you stay on track!